Georgenes Medeiros

Mental Health and the Internet:
6 Tips for Taking Care of Yourself

The Challenges of the Digital Age

2

Edition

English

Mental Health and the Internet:

6 Tips to Take Care of Yourself

**Georgenes Medeiros -
Second Edition**

ABOUT THE EDITOR

Georgenes Medeiros is Brazilian, graduated in Business Administration from Estácio de Sá College. He began working in the research field for editing and publishing digital content in 2018.

The author uses artificial intelligence to study and edit digital content for different platforms and social networks. There's no intention of plagiarism or copying original content. For those who are interested, I am available to provide assistance and freelance work on projects. Regarding the copyright of the editing, they are registered with the competent authorities in the region where they originated.

Introduction:

We live in a digital era where the internet plays a fundamental role in our lives. However, excessive and inappropriate internet usage can have significant impacts on our mental health. In this ebook, we will explore the relationship between mental health and the online world, providing 6 valuable tips to help you take care of your well-being while using the internet.

In the digital age, the internet stands as an invisible thread that weaves our lives into a complex web of connections. It stitches the narrative of our time, uniting continents and hearts with a keystroke. Through its virtual fibers, information flows like an incessant river, filling our minds with the knowledge of the world.

The internet offers us a world of wonders and possibilities. It connects us to people we could never have imagined meeting, allows us to share stories and experiences, and grants us access to a vast realm of information. Through it, we can learn, grow, and expand our horizons in ways that were once unimaginable.

However, this same powerful tool also casts its shadow. While it connects us virtually, it often disconnects us from the present. The glow of screens can obscure the beauty of real-world experiences, distancing us from the sensory richness that offline life offers. The constant pressure to share moments can lead us to value the image more than the experience itself.

As we deeply engage with the internet, the line between the real and the virtual often becomes blurred. The relentless pursuit of online validation can create a cycle of constant approval seeking, undermining our inner confidence. The continuous flow of information can flood our minds with anxiety, preventing us from finding calm.

Amidst this duality, we encounter a challenge: balancing the internet's unlimited potential with our emotional well-being. We need to navigate the digital waters with caution, reminding ourselves that we are human beings seeking genuine connection, not just online profiles. The key lies in finding harmony between the virtual world and the real world, where the internet is a tool that enhances our lives rather than dominates them.

As the digital era unfolds before us, it's important to remember that we are the captains of our own journeys. We can embrace the treasures of the internet while safeguarding our peace of mind. After all, the true value of life resides in authentic experience, real connections, and tangible emotions that we can only find in the world beyond the screens.

Chapter 1: Challenges of the Digital Era

In this chapter, we will address the challenges that the digital era presents to our mental health. From the pressure of social networks to constant online connectivity, we will discuss how these factors can affect our minds and emotions.

Living in the digital era has brought forth a series of challenges that directly impact our mental health. These challenges stem from the rapid and constant changes that technology has brought into our lives, primarily through the internet and social networks. Below, we will discuss some of the key challenges faced:

1. Pressure from Social Networks: Social networks have become an integral part of our online life, allowing us to share moments, opinions, and interact with others. However, the quest for validation through likes, comments, and followers can create a constant pressure to maintain a perfect image and an apparently ideal life. This can lead to feelings of inadequacy, anxiety, and even depression.

2. Constant Comparison: Constant exposure to the seemingly perfect lives of others on social networks can lead to comparison and the feeling that our own life is not as good as others'. This comparison can undermine self-esteem and generate feelings of dissatisfaction.

3. Information Overload: The amount of information available on the internet is staggering, but it can also be overwhelming. Constant exposure to negative news, conflicting information, and heated debates can cause anxiety and mental fatigue.

4. Technological Dependence: Excessive dependence on electronic devices and the internet can lead to distancing from real-world social interactions. This can result in isolation, impairing our ability to establish and maintain meaningful relationships.

5. Lack of Privacy: With the ease of online sharing, privacy has become a constant concern. The fear of personal information being exposed or used inappropriately can generate stress and anxiety.

6. FOMO (Fear of Missing Out): The sensation that we're missing out on something important when we're not online all the time can lead to a compulsion to constantly check social networks and stay connected. This can be exhausting and detrimental to our well-being.

7. Impact on Personal Relationships: Virtual communication can often replace personal interactions, affecting the quality of our relationships.

Electronic device addiction can cause us to ignore people around us and hinder the building of genuine connections.

In summary, the challenges of the digital era are related to social pressure, information overload, technological dependence, and the impact on our relationships. Recognizing and addressing these challenges is essential for maintaining balanced mental health and ensuring that the internet is a positive tool in our lives.

Chapter 2: Recognizing Warning Signs

It is essential to know how to recognize the warning signs that indicate mental health issues related to internet use. We will explore behavioral changes, such as social isolation, irritability, and anxiety, that may indicate the need to care for your mental well-being.

Excessive and inappropriate internet use can have a significant negative impact on our mental health. It is crucial to be attentive to the warning signs that indicate our relationship with the internet is affecting our emotional well-being. Here are some warning signs to watch out for:

1. Behavioral Changes: If you notice abrupt changes in your behavior, such as sudden social isolation, increased irritability, constant sadness, or changes in sleep patterns, this may be a sign that internet use is affecting your mental health.

2. Difficulty Disconnecting: Feeling constantly drawn to the screen of your device, even when you should be engaging in other important activities or interacting with people in the real world, can indicate problematic internet dependence.

3. Decline in Academic or Professional Performance: If you observe a significant drop in your academic or work performance, it could be related to excessive internet use. Frequent online procrastination may be an indication of mental health issues.

4. Social Isolation: Prioritizing online time over in-person interactions with friends and family can lead to social isolation, which in turn can negatively impact your mental health.

5. Anxiety and Depression: Persistent feelings of anxiety, deep sadness, hopelessness, or a lack of interest in activities that used to bring pleasure may be signs that the internet is negatively affecting your mental health.

6. Lack of Concentration: Difficulty staying focused on important tasks due to constant notifications checking, random internet browsing, or excessive online multitasking can indicate a problematic relationship with technology.

7. Impaired Self-Image and Self-Esteem: If internet use is leading you to constantly compare your life and appearance to others online, resulting in low self-esteem and feelings of inadequacy, this can be a concerning sign.

8. General Dissatisfaction:
Chronically feeling dissatisfied with your own life, often in comparison to the lives of others online, may indicate that internet use is harming your overall perspective and happiness.

Recognizing these warning signs is the first step in taking action to protect your mental health. If you notice that you are experiencing some of these signs, it is important to seek support, talk to friends, family, or mental health professionals, and consider adjusting your relationship with the internet to ensure you are taking good care of yourself.

Chapter 3: Establishing Healthy Boundaries

Setting boundaries is crucial for preserving your mental health. In this chapter, we will discuss the importance of defining internet usage schedules, regularly disconnecting, and setting clear limits on time spent in online activities.

Living in the digital era means being constantly connected and exposed to a multitude of online stimuli. However, setting boundaries is essential to maintain your mental health in balance. Here are some reasons why establishing boundaries is so crucial:

1. Prevention of Overwhelm:
Unlimited internet access can lead to information and stimulus overload. Setting limits on online time helps to avoid the feeling of being constantly bombarded with information, which can generate anxiety and stress.

2. Time for Important Activities:
Setting boundaries allows you to allocate time for activities that are important for your mental health, such as physical exercise, reading, meditation, or spending time with loved ones. This helps maintain a healthy balance between online and offline activities.

3. Improvement in Sleep Quality:
Excessive exposure to the blue light emitted by electronic devices can interfere with sleep quality. By setting limits on device usage before bedtime, you can improve your sleep and, consequently, your mental health.

4. Focus and Productivity:
Establishing specific schedules for internet usage helps improve focus and productivity in important tasks. By avoiding constant distractions, you can accomplish your activities more efficiently and feel a sense of achievement.

5. Preservation of Personal Relationships: Setting boundaries is also essential for maintaining healthy relationships. By reserving time for personal and in-person interactions, you strengthen your social and emotional bonds, which are vital for your mental health.

6. Stress Reduction: Excessive internet use can increase stress levels, especially when there's constant pressure to always be available online. Setting boundaries helps reduce stress related to time spent in online activities.

7. Self-Control and Self-Discipline: By setting boundaries, you develop important self-control and self-discipline skills. This can extend to other areas of your life, contributing to a sense of empowerment and overall well-being.

In summary, establishing healthy boundaries for internet usage is essential to protect your mental health. This allows you to be in control of your relationship with technology, avoiding its negative effects while enjoying its benefits. Remember that balance is key to a healthy digital life.

Chapter 4: Cultivating Meaningful Relationships

Social networks can connect us, but they can also leave us feeling isolated. We will address how to build meaningful relationships both online and offline to strengthen your support network and improve your mental health.

In an increasingly digitally connected world, building meaningful relationships is crucial in both online and offline environments. These relationships provide emotional support, social connections, and a sense of belonging. Here's the importance of cultivating these bonds in both contexts:

1. Online Relationships:

Building online relationships offers the opportunity to connect with people from different parts of the world and share common interests. These relationships can be enriching, allowing for exchanges of ideas, learning, and emotional support.

Expanding Social Networks:
Social networks provide a platform to connect with friends, family, and even meet new people with similar interests. This can expand your social network and introduce diverse perspectives.

Support in Online Communities:
Online groups and forums dedicated to specific topics offer an environment where you can find support and advice from people who share your interests or challenges.

2. Offline Relationships:

Offline relationships are essential for developing deep and authentic connections. They are built on face-to-face interactions, verbal communication, and direct human contact.

Deep Emotional Interactions: Face-to-face relationships allow for the expression of emotions and the creation of genuine connections that go beyond what is possible in online interactions.

Building Trust: Direct interaction with friends, family, and colleagues in the real world contributes to building trust, which is essential for forming lasting relationships.

Sharing Experiences:
Participating in offline activities such as social gatherings, cultural events, and sports provides shared experiences that strengthen bonds.

3. Balancing Online and Offline:

Finding the balance between online and offline relationships is essential for overall well-being. Both types of relationships have their own value and contribute to different aspects of your life.

Complementarity: Online relationships can complement offline ones, providing new perspectives and opportunities for connection.

Quality Time: By reserving time for offline in-person interactions, you create meaningful moments that cannot be replicated online.

Awareness and Limits: Stay mindful of the need to limit time spent online to ensure you are fully enjoying offline interactions.

Building meaningful relationships both online and offline is fundamental for your mental health and emotional well-being. Each type of relationship offers unique benefits, and finding a healthy balance between these two worlds helps ensure you are connected in an authentic and enriching way.

Chapter 5: Practicing Digital Self-Care

Digital self-care involves adopting practices that promote online well-being. We will explore mindfulness techniques, regular breaks, and the importance of consuming positive content to maintain a healthy mindset.

Digital self-care refers to conscious and healthy practices we adopt while interacting with the online world, aiming to protect our mental and emotional health. In the current digital landscape, where we are constantly connected and exposed to a variety of stimuli, digital self-care has become essential to preserving our well-being. Here are some key aspects of digital self-care:

1. Awareness of Online Time: Being aware of the time you spend online is the first step in digital self-care. This involves monitoring how much time you dedicate to online activities and evaluating whether it's affecting other areas of your life.

2. Regular Breaks: Taking regular breaks during internet usage is crucial to avoid fatigue and overwhelm. Set intervals where you disconnect completely, allowing your mind to rest and recover.

3. Conscious Content Consumption: Carefully select the type of content you consume online. Avoid excessive exposure to negative news or toxic content. Opt for information that enriches your mind and inspires positivity.

4. Mindfulness Practices: Apply mindfulness practices while browsing the internet. This involves being aware of your mental and emotional state as you engage online. Pay attention to your thoughts and emotions and take steps to avoid excessive distraction.

5. Set Clear Boundaries: Establish clear boundaries for internet usage. This includes setting specific times for checking emails, social media, and other online activities. Avoid the habit of constantly checking devices.

6. Disconnect Before Sleep: Avoid using electronic devices at least an hour before bedtime. The blue light emitted by screens can affect your sleep cycle, impacting your rest quality.

7. Prioritize Activities: Evaluate which online activities are truly important and prioritize them. Avoid the feeling of being constantly connected to all platforms and apps.

8. Beware of Social Comparison: Remember that online life often presents idealized versions of reality. Avoid comparing your life to what is shared on social media.

9. Seek Positive Inspiration: Look for online content that is inspiring, educational, and motivating. Follow profiles and pages that promote positivity and personal growth.

10. Set Device Limits: Define time limits for electronic device usage, especially for non-essential activities. Use apps and settings that help you monitor and limit time spent on specific apps.

Digital self-care is a proactive approach to dealing with the challenges of the digital era. By adopting these practices, you can harness the benefits of technology while safeguarding your mental and emotional health. Remember that balance is key, and digital self-care is a powerful tool to achieve it.

Chapter 6: Seeking Professional Help

If you're facing significant mental health challenges, it's important to seek professional help. We will discuss how to identify when it's time to seek a mental health professional and how therapy can be beneficial.

Facing significant mental health challenges is a complex and often challenging journey, involving dealing with emotional, psychological, and behavioral issues that negatively impact a person's mental well-being. These challenges can vary in severity and nature, encompassing a wide range of mental health conditions. Here are some key points about addressing these challenges:

1. Recognition and Acceptance: The first step is to recognize that you're facing mental health challenges and to accept that it's part of your journey. Denial or stigma surrounding mental health can delay the process of seeking help.

2. Seeking Professional Help: In many cases, dealing with significant mental health challenges requires the intervention of mental health professionals such as psychologists, psychiatrists, therapists, and counselors. These experts are trained to provide guidance, diagnosis, and appropriate treatment.

3. Therapy and Treatment: Therapy is a crucial approach to addressing mental health challenges. Different types of therapy, such as cognitive-behavioral therapy, talk therapy, or group therapy, may be recommended based on individual needs.

4. Medication Use: In some cases, the use of medication prescribed by a psychiatrist may be necessary to manage severe mental health symptoms such as depression, anxiety, or bipolar disorder. It's important to strictly follow medical guidance.

5. Support Network: Having a support network composed of friends, family, and loved ones is essential. These individuals can offer emotional support, understanding, and encouragement throughout the coping process.

6. Ongoing Self-Care:
Consistently practicing self-care, including physical exercise, healthy eating, adequate sleep, and relaxation techniques, can help strengthen your emotional resilience.

7. Mental Health Education:
Understanding your mental health condition, its symptoms, and possible treatments is crucial. Education helps demystify mental health and make informed decisions about your well-being.

8. Patience and Persistence:
Facing significant mental health challenges is an ongoing process that requires patience and persistence. Improvement can be gradual and vary from person to person.

9. Avoiding Isolation: Staying connected with others and avoiding social isolation is crucial. Isolating yourself can worsen symptoms and make seeking help more difficult.

10. Setting Small Goals: Establishing realistic and achievable goals can help promote a sense of accomplishment and progress along the recovery journey.

Facing significant mental health challenges is a courageous step toward your own well-being. Remember that you're not alone on this journey and that support is available to help you overcome difficulties and build a healthier, more balanced life.

Conclusion:

The internet is a powerful tool that can impact our mental health in various ways. By adopting the tips presented in this ebook, you will be better equipped to face the challenges of the digital age while actively taking care of your mental well-being. Remember that balance between the online world and personal care is essential to live a fulfilling and healthy life.

The internet is a fascinating and dynamic world, stretching before us like a vast ocean of possibilities. A tool that, while bringing numerous advantages and conveniences, also holds a profound influence over our mental health. Its threads of connection reach our hearts and minds, shaping our perception of the world and ourselves.

Through social media, we find friends, share moments, and maintain bonds even across distances. Yet, beneath the veil of likes and comments, subtle traps of comparison hide, nurturing seeds of self-doubt and anxiety. The pursuit of virtual validation often distances us from true human connection, sowing loneliness amid a digital crowd.

The torrent of information that the internet offers, while being a feast of knowledge, can overwhelm our minds with impactful news, conflicting opinions, and incessant debates. Constant exposure to negativity can create a fog of despair, obscuring our view of the beauty and positivity that exist in the world.

The boundaries of time disappear when we're online. Screen addiction can envelop us in a constant digital embrace, blurring the lines between work and leisure, day and night. This incessant connection, while a boon for immediate information, can also be a curse to our inner peace and rest.

However, just as the waves of the internet can rock our emotional boat, we can also learn to navigate wisely. We can consciously choose what we consume online, selecting emotional nutrients over virtual toxins. We can set limits to protect our attention and inner peace, allowing us to disconnect in order to reconnect with the present.

The internet is undoubtedly a double-edged sword. If we wield its blades with gentleness and discernment, it can become a powerful ally in our journey for mental health. It's up to each of us to cultivate a healthy relationship with this tool, remembering that at the core of it all, our mental health is a precious gem that deserves to be protected and nurtured with love and care.

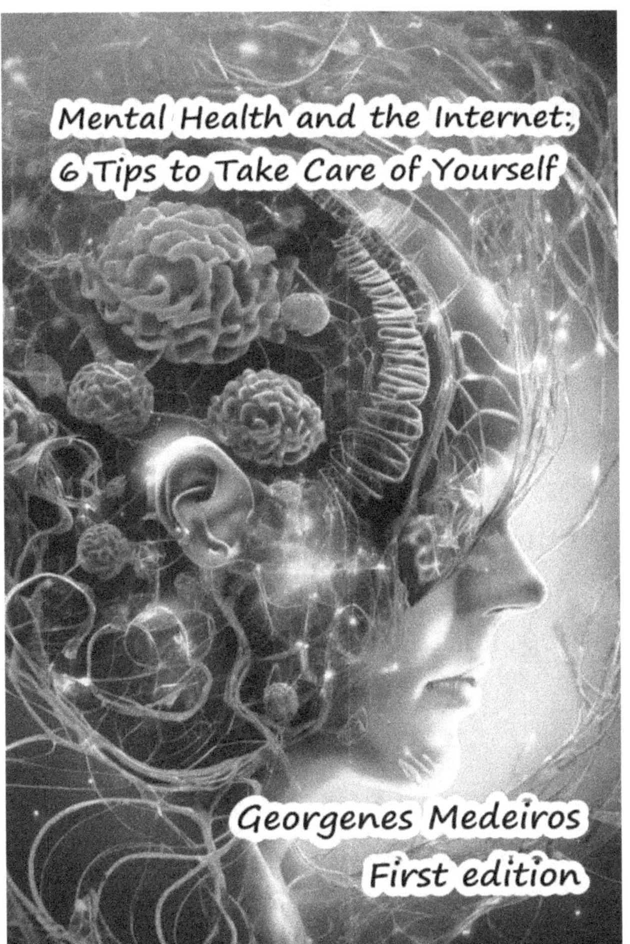

Mental Health and the Internet:
6 Tips to Take Care of Yourself
Georgenes Medeiros
First edition

Mental Health and the Internet: 6 Tips for Taking Care of Yourself

Editing: Georgenes Medeiros

Copyright © 2024

9 798878 414548